The Wonders Of Tea Tree Oil

Remedies And Recipes Included

By

Gene Ashburner

ISBN-13:978-1508776772
ISBN-10:1508776776

Content

Tea Tree Oil

Melaleuca oil or tea tree oil as it is also known, is a pale yellow essential oil that has a camphoraceous aroma. It is a natural antiseptic that is effective as an antibiotic, anti-viral and fungicide.

Melaleuca oil or tea tree oil may be applied full strength or diluted in water or other type of oil like olive oil.

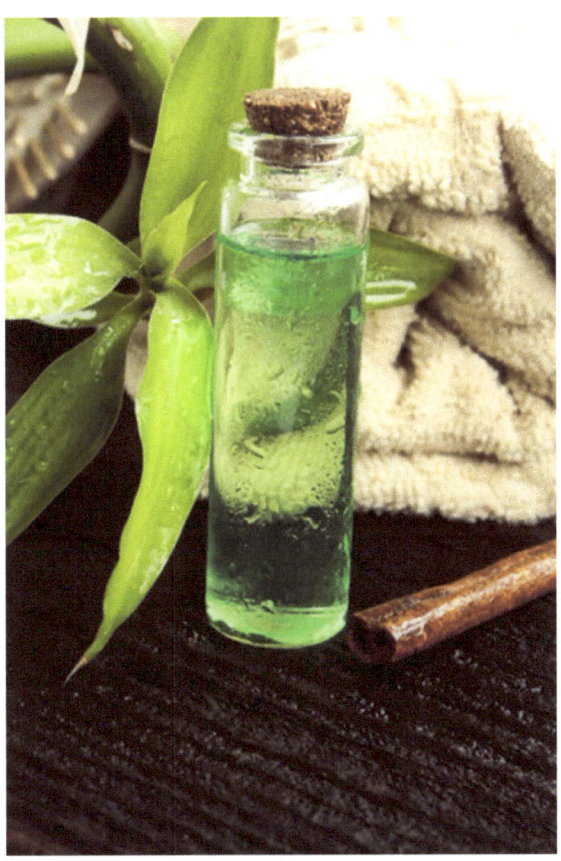

How Is Tea Tree Oil Made

Tea tree oil is oil made from the leaves of the Melaleuca alternifolia tree. These trees are found on the north-east coast of New South Wales in Australia.

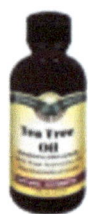 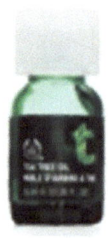 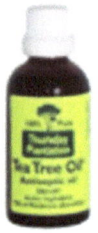

Examples Of Tea Tree Oil On The Market

Diluting Tea Tree Oil

You can dilute tea tree oil with carrier oils such as:

- ❖ Olive oil
- ❖ Grapeseed oil
- ❖ Sweet almond oil
- ❖ Coconut oil
- ❖ Jojoba oil

You can also dilute tea tree oil with a neutral cream, gel, lotion or ointment.

Note:

Diluted tea tree oil should be stored in a cool dark place and should not be stored for longer than 3 months.

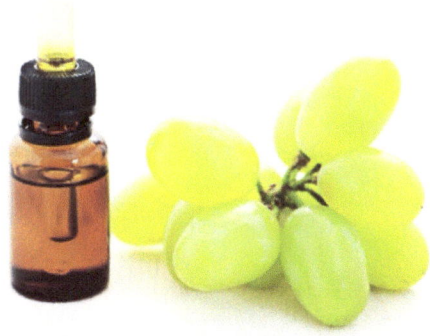

Grapeseed Oil

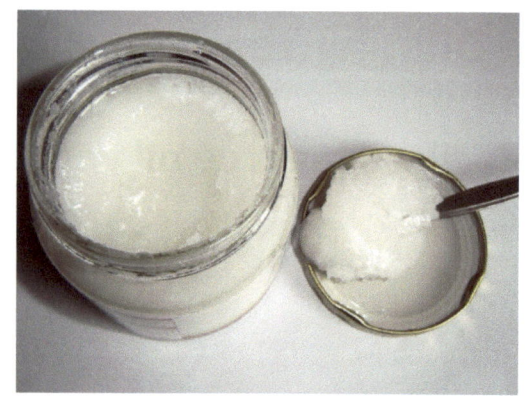

Coconut Oil

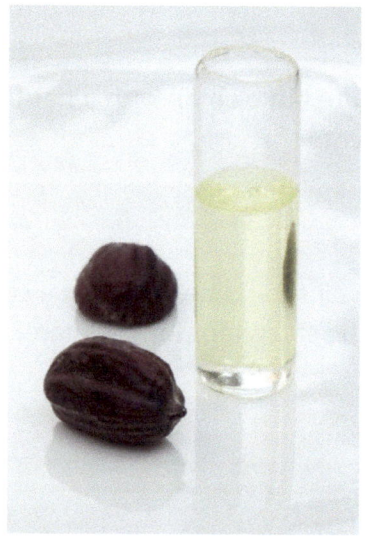

Jojoba Oil

There Are Many Uses For Tree Tea Oil

There are many external uses for tea tree oil but it should not be taken internally:

Tea tree oil is often used in topical mixtures to help fight bacterial infections.

- ❖ Acne
- ❖ Antiseptic
- ❖ Arthritis / Rheumatism Relief
- ❖ Athletes Foot Remedy
- ❖ Boils
- ❖ Bruises And Burns
- ❖ Chest Congestion
- ❖ Cold Sores
- ❖ Dandruff
- ❖ Hair Lice
- ❖ Haemorrhoids Relief
- ❖ Insect Repellent
- ❖ Itchy Remedy
- ❖ Mold Removal
- ❖ Oral Care

- ❖ Remedy To Remove Ticks
- ❖ Sinus Remedy
- ❖ Sunburn Remedy
- ❖ Toe Fungus Removal
- ❖ Wart Removal
- ❖ Yeast Infections

Health Remedies

Acne Remedy

Ingredients

>   100 ml Aloe Vera gel
>
>   5 ml tea tree oil

Method

Combine the Aloe Vera gel and tea tree oil together.

Mix well.

Store in a dark glass bottle.

Use as face wash.

Antiseptic Remedy

Tea tree oil has properties that will sanitize, heal cuts and wounds and ease pain.

Tea tree oil is great for oral care and will calm the sores in your mouth and gums.

Ingredients

>   10 ml lavender oil
>
>   10 ml tea tree oil

Method

Combine the lavender oil and tea tree oil together.

Mix well.

Pour the mixture into a dark bottle.

Pour a few drops of the mixture into the water when cleaning the wounds or you can apply the tea tree oil mixture directly to the gauze or bandage before applying it onto the wound.

Arthritis / Rheumatism Relief

Sweet Almond Oil Remedy

Ingredients

36 drops tea tree oil

62,5 ml sweet almond oil

Method

Combine the tea tree oil and sweet almond oil together.

Mix well.

Pour the mixture into a dark glass bottle.

Apply 3 to 4 times per day.

Note:

Store the mixture in a dark bottle.

Pure Tea Tree Oil Remedy

Ingredients

Few drops tea tree oil

Method

Drop a few drops of tea tree oil into a bath of warm water. Lie and soak in the bath to alleviate the joint pain.

Athletes Foot Remedy

Ingredients

20 to 30 drops tea tree oil

Warm water

Method

Add the tea tree oil drops to a small bowl of warm water. Soak the feet in the warm water mixture 20 minutes. Repeat 3 times daily.

Boil Remedy

Ingredients

Tea tree oil

Cotton cloth

Gauze

Damp washcloth

Dry towel

Heating pad

Method

Drip the tea tree oil onto a cotton cloth and dab onto the boil.

Cover the boil with a piece of gauze.

Cover the gauze with a damp washcloth.

Then replace the damp washcloth with a dry towel.

Then replace the dry towel with a heating pad left on for 15 minutes.

Repeat the process (this will bring the boil to the surface of the skin).

Bruises And Burns Remedy

Ingredients

Few drops tea tree oil

Few drops lavender oil

Method

Combine a few drops of tea tree oil and lavender oil together.

Mix well.

Pour the mixture into a dark glass bottle.

Rub the oil mixture onto the bruises or burns.

Chest Congestion Remedy

Add a few drops of tea tree oil to a vaporizer to help loosen a congested chest.

Cold Sore Remedy

Tea tree oil helps to numb cold sores in a similar way that menthol does.

Rub the tea tree oil directly onto the cold sore.

Dandruff Remedy 1

Ingredients

Tea tree oil

Method

Massage the tea tree oil into the scalp.

Leave for 1 hour.

Rinse out with shampoo and warm water.

Dandruff Remedy 2

Ingredients

16 fluid ounces mild shampoo

20 drops tea tree oil

Method

Combine the shampoo and tea tree oil together.

Mix well.

Pour into a dark glass bottle.

Use as an ordinary shampoo.

Dandruff Remedy 3

Ingredients

50 ml tea tree oil

50 ml evening primrose oil

Method

Combine the Tea Tree oil and evening primrose oil together.

Mix well.

Rub the oil mixture directly onto the scalp.

Leave overnight.

Rinse out with warm water.

Dandruff Remedy 4

Ingredients

50 ml tea tree oil

50 ml flaxseed oil

Method

Combine the Tea Tree oil and flaxseed oil together.

Mix well.

Rub the oil mixture directly onto the scalp.

Leave overnight.

Rinse out with warm water.

Hair Lice Removal Remedy

Ingredients

125 ml coconut shampoo

125 ml tea tree oil

Method

Combine the coconut shampoo and tea tree oil together.

Mix well.

Lather the shampoo mixture into the hair.

Cover the head with plastic or a shower cap.

Leave for 120 minutes.

Rinse the shampoo off the hair with warm water.

Apply coconut conditioner onto the hair.

Comb the hair with a nit comb.

Do this 3 times a week for 2 weeks.

Hemorrhoids Relief

Ingredients

Tea tree oil

Method

Use as an astringent directly onto the affected area.

Insect Repellent

Ingredients

60 drops tea tree oil

15 ml coconut oil.

Method

Combine the tea tree oil and coconut oil together.

Mix well.

Pour the mixture into a dark glass bottle.

Rub the mixture onto the skin to prevent insect bites.

Itch Relief Remedy

Ingredients

12,5 ml undiluted tea tree oil

25 ml glycerine

56 ml Aloe Vera juice

Method

Combine the tea tree oil and glycerine together.

Mix well.

Add the Aloe Vera juice.

Mix well.

Pour the mixture into a spray bottle.

Store in a dark place.

Spray onto affected itchy areas when necessary.

Oral Care With Tea Tree Oil

Tea tree oil prevents plaque build up and tooth decay.

It is ideal for maintaining oral hygiene, dentures, bad breath, tartar build up and gum health.

Tea tree oil helps reduce bad breath.

Remedy To Remove Ticks

Ingredients

Few drops of pure tea tree oil

Method

Drop the tea tree oil directly onto the tick, this will make the tick unlatch from the skin.

Sinus Remedy

Ingredients

Few drops tea tree oil

Boiling water

Method

Pour a few drops on tea tree oil into a bowl of boiling water.

Hold your face over the steaming bowl with a towel thrown over your head.

Do this for about 15 minutes and you will feel a big difference in your sinuses.

Do this at least 3 times per day.

Sunburn Remedy 1

Ingredients

50 ml coconut oil

5 ml tea tree oil

Method

Combine the coconut oil and tea tree oil together.

Mix well.

Apply the mixture to the affected sunburned areas.

Sunburn Remedy 2

Ingredients

Tea tree oil (undiluted)

Method

Apply undiluted tea tree oil to the affected sunburned areas.

Note:

Undiluted tea tree oil can sometimes irritate a person's skin; make sure you are not one of these people. Test the undiluted tea tree oil on a very small portion of your skin first.

Sunburn Remedy 3

Ingredients

7,5 drops tea tree oil

16 drops lavender oil

4 oz distilled water

Method

Combine the tea tree oil, lavender oil and distilled water together.

Mix well.

Pour the mixture into a spray bottle.

Spray the affected sunburned areas.

Sunburn Remedy 4

Ingredients

10 drops tea tree oil

25 ml Aloe Vera lotion

Method

Combine the tea tree oil and Aloe Vera lotion together.

Mix well.

Apply the mixture to the affected sunburned areas.

Toe Fungus Remedy

Ingredients

Few drops Tea Tree Oil

Method

Apply a few drops of tea tree oil directly onto the infected toenail.

Rub the tea tree oil into the top of the nail as well as under the nail.

Repeat 1 time per day.

Wart Removal remedy

Dab the diluted tea tree oil onto the wart. You can dilute the tea tree oil with carrier oil – see section on Diluting Tea Tree Oil.

Yeast Infection Remedy

Ingredients

    1 Tampon

    Olive oil

    Few drops Tea Tree Oil

Method

Coat the top of the tampon with olive oil.

Drop a few drops of tea tree oil onto the tampon.

Insert the tampon into the vagina.

Household Uses For Tea Tree Oil

Mold Remover Remedy

Ingredients

Water

Few drops tea tree oil

Method

Drop a few drops of tea tree oil into the water.

Mix well.

Wipe down the affected areas with the tea tree oil and water mixture.

The tea tree oil will inhibit the mold from growing.

Tea Tree Room Spray

Tea tree oil is an odor neutralizer so is ideal to use in room sprays.

Ingredients

250 ml water

250 ml pure lemon juice

Few drops tea tree oil

Method

Combine the water, lemon juice and tea tree oil together.

Mix well.

Pour the mixture into a spray bottle.

Spray the room with the mixture when the room needs to be freshened.

Tea Tree Oil Used For Pets

Tea tree oil can be used for bites, cuts, stings, rashes, dermatitis, lice, mange, ringworm, fleas and ticks.

Diluted solutions of tea tree oil can be as a remedy to treat bacterial and fungal infections in aquarium fish.

Skin Conditions In Dogs

Combine a few drops of tea tree oil into the dog shampoo.

This will treat itching and non specific skin conditions in dogs.

Ear Infections In Dogs

Insert small amounts of tea tree oil into the dog's ear; this will kill the bacteria that cause the ear infection.

Side Effects Of Tea Tree Oil

Pregnant and breastfeeding women should avoid using tea tree oil.

Undiluted tea tree oil could cause itchiness, irritation, and redness on skin, test a small portion of your skin before applying it to larger areas!

Never drink pure tea tree oil as it could cause diarrhoea, vomiting, impaired immune function, excessive drowsiness, sleepiness, confusion, poor coordination and coma.

Never allow pure tea tree oil near the eyes, genitals or mouth.

Tea Tree Oil Warnings

Tea tree oil is for EXTERNAL USE ONLY.

Avoid contact with eyes when using tea tree oil.

Do not apply tea tree oil to broken or irritated skin.

Do not use tea tree oil on sensitive skin.

Always keep the tea tree oil in a dry place (and a dark bottle).

Tea tree oil contains amounts of 1,8 cineole which is a skin irritant, test a small portion of your skin before applying it to larger areas

Tea tree oil is considered safe for external use for most adults but beware of just using it on children.

Recipes

Tea Tree Oil Wash

Ingredients

15 ml sea salt

12 drops tea tree oil

580 ml warm water

Method

Combine the sea salt, tea tree oil and warm water together.

Mix until the salt has dissolved.

Pour into a spray bottle and spray the mixture onto the affected areas.

Tea Tree Deodorant

Ingredients

125 ml coconut oil

166 ml baking soda

250 ml arrowroot powder

25 drops tea tree oil

Method

Place the coconut oil into a heat proof bowl.

Place the bowl over boil water for a minute or two until the coconut oil has melted.

Remove the coconut oil from the heat and set aside to cool but not set.

Add the baking soda, arrowroot powder and tea tree oil.

Mix well.

Store in a sealed dark glass container.

Disinfectant Hand Wash

Ingredients

20 to 30 drops tea tree oil

250 ml fragrance free liquid soap

Method

Combine the tea tree oil and the liquid soap together.

Mix well.

Decant the liquid soap mixture into a soap dispenser bottle.

Use as normal liquid hand wash soap.

Baby Wipes

Ingredients

62,5 ml Aloe Vera juice

4 drops lavender oil

62,5 ml water

2 drops tea tree oil

1/2 roll paper towels (cut lengthwise)

Method

Combine the Aloe Vera juice, lavender oil, water and tea tree oil together.

Mix well.

Place the paper towels into a plastic container.

Pour the liquid mixture over the paper towels.

Seal the container.

Use as standard wet wipes.

Tea Tree Oil And Green Tea Skin Toner

Ingredients

1 green tea teabag

125 ml boiling water

4 drops tea tree oil

Method

Steep the teabag in the boiling water for 2 to 3 minutes.

Remove the tea bag.

Allow the water cool.

Add the tea tree oil.

Mix well.

Pour the cooled mixture into a bottle.

Use with cotton pads like you would regular toner.

Tea Tree Oil Toothpaste

Ingredients

18 ml coconut oil

56 ml bicarbonate of soda

18 ml sea salt

7 drops mint oil

8 drops tea tree oil

Method

Place the coconut oil in a heatproof bowl over a bowl of boiling water.

Once the coconut oil has melted remove from the heat and set aside to cool down BUT NOT SET.

Add the bicarbonate of soda, salt, peppermint oil and tea tree oil.

Mix well.

Store the mixture in a dark glass jar.

Use as normal toothpaste.

Massage Oil Recipe

Ingredients

40 ml grape seed oil

6 drops jasmine oil

2 drops tea tree oil

2 drops Neroli oil

Method

Combine the grape seed oil, jasmine oil, tea tree oil and Neroli oil together.

Mix well.

Pour the mixture into a dark glass bottle.

Before application warm the oil.